UNLOCKING WEIGHT LOSS

HOW TO NAVIGATE ROADBLOCKS TO ACHIEVE YOUR GOALS

By: The Wellness Preacher

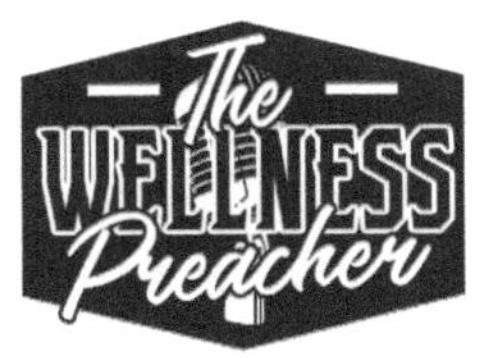

Unlocking Weight Loss
How to Navigate Roadblocks to Achieve Your Goals

Printed in the United States of America

Author: Qaadir'Naqib Muhammad

ISBN: 979-8-9903974-5-3

Published by: Ahvision Publishing
Edited and Book Cover Design
www.ahvisionpublishing.com

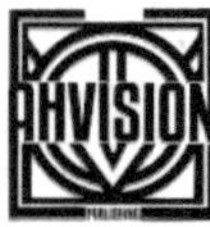

TABLE OF CONTENTS

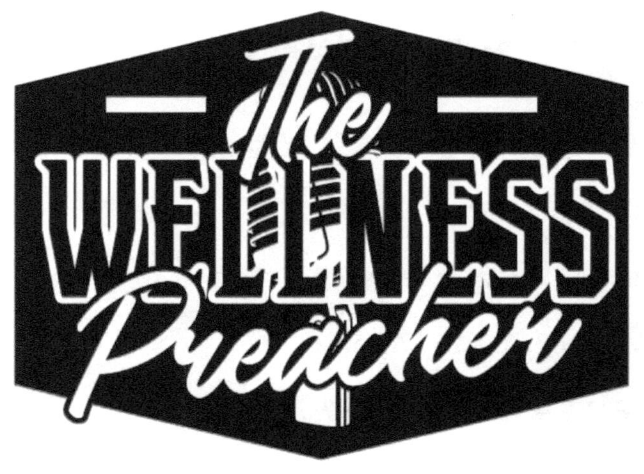

www.TheWellnessPreacher.com
IG: @thewellnesspreacher

IN HONOR OF

This book is in honor of my little brother, Malachi Elijah Muhammad. I originally published it on February 9, 2018, marking the one-year anniversary of his transition from this dimensional reality to another on February 9, 2017. There's no worse feeling than losing someone close to you who lives under the same roof. I had shared with my brother my desire to release my first book within the year, and little did I know that his death would become my inspiration to make it happen.

The biggest factor and inspiration that led to the decision to publish on the day of his transition was the pain I felt on his birthday, January 3rd, knowing that February 9th was the next month. I didn't want to experience that pain back-to-back, so I decided to change the meaning and memory of that day, not just for myself but for my family as well. God willing, this day will be remembered as the day one of our family members became a published author rather than the day we lost a loved one.

Malachi was more than just my little brother; he became my accountability partner in many areas of my life. As Muslims, we are taught to pray five times a day, and my brother did so daily and then some. Although I could not pray alongside him five times a day due to our schedules, there was one time of day when we made sure to pray together: our morning prayer at 5 a.m. As he led the prayer, I would listen and repeat silently. One thing that always stood out to me was that he always asked Allah to cover the brotherhood and sisterhood and to unite the Muslim world.

After a while, Malachi became my workout partner. After prayer, he would ask me, "Are we going to the gym tonight?" I would say, "Yes, sir." Later, he came into my room and asked, "Are we still going to the gym?" I replied regretfully, "Sure, give me a few minutes." About an hour went by, and he came back and asked, "Are you tired, bro?" I said, "Yes, sir," thinking he would say, "It's cool, we can go tomorrow." However, instead, he said, "If you don't get up, I'm changing your name to Mr. EXCUSES instead of Mr. NO EXCUSES and taking your G-card away from you." We smiled and laughed, then I got up, and we went to work out.

FOREWORD

By Bilal Munir Rahim

Let's talk about excitement. I am extremely excited that my brother and author of this book, Qaadir Naqib Muhammad, has reached this point in his journey. What a milestone to celebrate! Qaadir and I have accomplished many goals during our short time of collaborating in business. I have watched him pursue and conquer his own personal goals as well, and that is why I constantly encouraged him to finish this book and tell his story.

It takes a lifetime to learn yourself because you are constantly changing. You should constantly be growing and evolving; therefore, if you pay attention to yourself, you can always learn something new. Personal development is a sensitive subject to most, especially when you haven't quite reached your goal. There is also a small group of people who are always willing to share their trials with others, hoping they can help prevent them from making the same mistakes. Trust me, I completely understand whichever category you fall under when discussing personal development.

When we are crushing our goals, we love to share that happy feeling with others, and when we are not doing so well, others will never know. Part of the reason for that is that we are protecting the motivation and overall mood of our peers. We should strive to make sure that the time we share with one another is positive and uplifting. Supporting your friends and family is important because you never know what insecurities they have overcome to reach the starting point.

In this book, you will learn that it is okay to fail and that it is okay to succeed. In each chapter, Qaadir invites us to experience the journey of weight loss along with him. This book will be a shocking reality for some, and for other readers, it will be just the confirmation needed. The tips and information presented here are for anyone who has ever set out to accomplish a goal.

Today, we are faced with the highest rates of childhood obesity that America has seen. Not to mention the statistics that 1 in 2 adults are also obese. The future of our existence depends on us staying fit and healthy. That means regular exercise and conscious eating habits. If you are reading this foreword, that means you have already taken a huge step in getting started. Congratulations! I would like to encourage you to dig deep, take notes, and commit yourself to becoming the best that you can be.

Bilal Munir Rahim

INTRODUCTION

"This material aims to share with you..."

INTRODUCTION

This material aims to share with you the struggles and lessons that come with becoming the best you can be in your lifetime. On this journey, I intend to inspire you to join me or allow me to join you so we can reach our destination together. Take the time to review each chapter as many times as you need to extract the lessons from my experiences thus far. You may uncover a lesson for yourself that I didn't notice and perhaps wasn't meant to notice at the time.

I originally wanted to wait until I reached a certain point in my weight goal before completing this book. I had what seemed like legitimate reasons, such as including images throughout the book and ending with a photo of me at my desired weight. However, it became clear that I should publish this work now. I needed to let go of the idea that I had to look a certain way before releasing this book and focus on the bigger picture instead of myself.

Each moment shared in this work is factual and actually took place in my life. Nothing has been changed or rearranged. As you embark on your journey to read this work, take some time to use the space provided at the end of this book to reflect and write about the areas you can improve, whether it involves adding something to your life or removing something. As you use that space, be open and honest; after all, you're writing to yourself about yourself, so why not? I hope that these words reach your heart and ignite your drive to push through to the next level.

CHAPTER 1

Is It My DNA?

"Three hundred thirty pounds..."

CHAPTER 1

Is It My DNA

Three hundred thirty pounds is what appeared on the scale before my eyes. In my mind, I could hear Jay-Z's voice saying, "Numbers don't lie," and reality kicked in at that moment. It was now or never; my health and well-being had become important to me. Reflecting on what I had attempted to do in the past to lose weight—this membership, that membership, these fees, and those fees—it became clear that going to the gym required a commitment that was not in sight at this time and would be a waste of funds that could be used elsewhere.

At that moment, the first step became clear to me: I needed to get in the habit of working out regularly without a financial obligation connected to it first. So here I go, my mind made up; this is my year to get the body I always wanted, and nobody is going to stop me. I found a park near my house with a walking trail and started walking it as often as possible. After a while, I was able to start mixing a little walking with a bit of jogging, and in my mind, I was doing GREAT! I could jog for a few yards and eventually got to the point where I could jog a whole lap around the trail without stopping.

Working out became a routine; it was mandatory that I walk every day, and if I didn't, my day just wouldn't be right. I was exercising and working on a committed relationship, and we enjoyed spending time together. During this time, I did not spend money on anything, from clothes to a scale.

I found an old pair of shoes in the closet, some sweatpants, and a shirt I didn't wear anymore, so I made that my walking gear. The thought of getting on a scale was on my mind, but the fear of seeing those numbers again kept me from getting on a scale, let alone purchasing one to haunt me in my own home. That was not an option.

After a few months, I started feeling the urge to jog more and more each time I went for my walk, and it was then that I understood it was okay to listen to what my body was striving to convey to me. My body was letting me know that it was time to go to the next level and that it needed more than just walking around and jogging. So, it was time to start investing in my wellness, which meant that getting a gym membership was not only okay but a requirement at this time. Plus, I was not able to track my progress; I still didn't have a scale, and I didn't even know how far I was walking on the trail.

As most of you know, whenever you sign up for a membership, they want to walk you around and tell you about what they have and how you can get it if you pay just a few more monthly dollars. So, when I walked in, I STOPPED the guy at the door the moment I walked in. My mind was set on just getting access to the equipment. I told the guy, "Please don't offer me anything else. I am not interested in a tour of your facility, sir. If it's okay with you, here is my identification and debit card. Can we just go straight to the paperwork?" I remember him looking at me to see if I was upset or in a rush, wondering if he should do what he had been trained to do or as the customer requested. After he decided to do what was asked of him, we had a great conversation while he made me a new member.

The next day, I was walking on the treadmill. Usually, I would walk a few laps at the park and thought that was enough. Now that I was in the gym, I could track my distance and time with the machine. I thought walking was sufficient since I just wanted to lose weight and wasn't focused on building muscle. I didn't ask anyone for advice because I believed that the weight would start to come off as long as I was walking. I couldn't be any more wrong.

After several months of consistent exercise, I stepped onto the scale. My clothes started feeling big on me, so I thought I must have lost some weight. Stepping on that scale can either make or break you. After stepping on it that first time, I realized I didn't know much about losing weight. Only running on a treadmill wasn't working fast enough. Don't get me wrong; I lost a few pounds, but after several months of hard work in the gym, it seemed there should have been more weight loss.

I realized it was crucial to start lifting weights and using different gym equipment. After all, that was why I was there—to use the equipment to lose weight. I became addicted to getting on the scale at the start and end of each workout to track my progress. This helped me understand what was working for my body. Finally, the pounds started fading away, and my confidence was building. I was excited to see the new numbers with each visit to the gym.

Then, one day, the numbers stopped changing. It became clear that I had reached a plateau. I needed to humble myself and get advice from a professional or find a mentor to help me get to the next level. During this time, I realized that men often don't ask for help when dealing with challenges. It became crystal clear that only fools refuse to see that they need help from an outside source.

Before I accepted that getting help was the best option, I made excuses like, "It's my metabolism," "I'm big-boned," "I didn't park far enough from the door," or "God is mad at me right now." Being in denial is our greatest enemy to progress in relationships, business, school, weight loss, and much more. After making one phone call to a brother with over twenty years of bodybuilding experience and applying his suggestions, the plateau was gone, and the pounds started fading away again.

Keys to remember:

1. Get in the habit of working out before making a financial commitment.
2. Don't spend any money until you've established a workout routine.
3. Wait until your body tells you it's time to go to the next level.
4. Put your pride and ego aside and speak to a professional.

CHAPTER 2

What is Stress?

"As long as we are alive, we will encounter..."

CHAPTER 2

Was It Stress?

As long as we are alive, we will encounter stress. In fact, each time we work out, we apply stress to our tendons and ligaments to build muscle and improve our health and well-being. After starting my journey to lose weight, it seemed like the stress committee had it out for me. Daily stress attacks were relentless, and I couldn't catch a break if my life depended on it. Eventually, going to the gym became a thing of the past; my time became limited, and I just didn't have time to work out. But I told myself that as things settled down, I would return to it harder than before.

Well, during this time, I broke my wrist and needed surgery. As you might guess, working out wasn't an option, giving me a legitimate excuse for not going to the gym. After surgery, the doctor told me I wouldn't be going to therapy. Instead, if I wanted to regain full motion and use of my wrist, I had to follow the exercises on the paper he handed me. The sheet only had images of hand exercises, no directions or instructions, just pictures. I tried my best to listen as he talked, but I remember holding back tears, thinking about my empty savings, upcoming rent, and already-spent funds. Then, the reality of managing our funds better started to set in. The feeling that I had let my family down was beating me up inside, applying stress like never before.

Now, I was at home recovering, unable to work because the medication caused drowsiness. And when you take strong meds, what do you usually do? Most likely, you guessed it right: EAT.

So there I was, lying in bed, unable to drive (which was how I made a living), eating, and taking pills to ease the pain. As you may already know, this is a recipe for weight gain. Each day, every hour on the hour, I diligently did the wrist exercises the doctor gave me, even doing them twice as often as recommended.

As this chapter of my life was closing and I was preparing to go back to work, the doctor asked me to get on the scale. When the numbers read 335 pounds, my heart dropped. It was then I realized that my wrist was broken, not my legs. The reality set in that if I wanted to keep the weight off, I just needed to watch what I was eating and walk around the house or at the gym since my membership was still active.

To be honest, there was a time I went to the gym to cancel or put my account on hold because of my injury. The manager told me I could still use the gym. I asked, "Do I need clearance from the doctor?" I remember his exact words: "You are an adult. If you feel like you can do it, do it. I don't need a doctor's note to tell me you can use a machine, but we will not be able to cancel or put your account on hold." I couldn't think of a response, so I said okay and walked out.

As I left the doctor's office, the manager's words came back to haunt me. I realized that stress did not bring the weight back, nor was it the reason I needed to lose weight in the first place. I then understood that although there are two types of stress, both are designed to make us better and stronger. The first form of stress comes without our input and is attached to life, meaning life gives us obstacles and roadblocks. Whether we like it or not, they come.

These roadblocks, also known as stress, are not designed to beat us down but rather to build us up and teach us lessons that will make us stronger. Then, we have the stress we do have control over, which occurs when we decide to exercise. Whether it's to lose weight, tone up, or build muscle, each involves applying stress to our bodies.

Keys to remember:

1. What can you do right now in your current situation?
2. Stress is designed to make you stronger and better.
3. Save money for unexpected loss of income. Create residual income for yourself.

CHAPTER 3

Are You Afraid?

"After being on this journey of..."

CHAPTER 3

Are You Afraid?

After being on this journey of losing weight, or as my brother likes to say, "enhancing the quality of your look," I had to ask myself what my problem was. A few years had come and gone, and a few pounds had come and gone, but mostly, they kept coming back. At this point, I had too much information about what to do and what not to do regarding enhancing the quality of my look. Once again, I was above three hundred pounds after getting down to two hundred and sixty at one point and maintaining it for a few months.

Having a heart-to-heart conversation with myself, I raised some questions: Are you afraid of how you will look? Do you think your head will be bigger than your body? These were just a few of the questions I asked myself. Having knowledge about something is good, but being able to execute it matters most. The knowledge worked because I gave it to other people who were using it to lose weight. So, it was time for this conversation to take place and for these questions to be answered by me, no one else.

Each time I reached a certain phase in my journey, different things would start happening that I wasn't used to. It's like giving a broken person love for the first time. Even though they might be looking for love, they usually reject it because it's foreign to them. As I was enhancing the quality of my look, the attention that came with it was foreign to me—not just attention from women, but simply standing out more when I was usually the invisible person at social functions, or at least that's how it seemed to me.

I did not grow up with confidence, and honestly, I don't even remember engaging in activities that would build my self-esteem or confidence as a young man. Becoming an adult without these characteristics has an impact. This is why it's important for us as parents and as a community to build each other up. We should refer each other to programs that address these issues within our community, especially for our youth. It is crucial for a young man to have confidence and feel good about himself.

Sometimes, I would see my reflection and recognize my progress, only to start gaining the weight back. This was insane, especially for someone who had worked hard to lose those pounds. I remember telling myself that it was easy for me to lose weight, so it wasn't a problem. But in reality, I was afraid to reach my weight goal. I was afraid of becoming the big guy who lost all that weight and now looks sick with a big head.

After having these discussions with myself, I decided it was time to put up or shut up. People are watching and encouraged when they see someone else succeed because it reminds them they can do it, too. If you can relate to these words, please understand that people are also watching you as I am still working on reaching my desired weight. All you have to do, like I did, is make it up in your mind to lose that weight and enhance the quality of your look. Take it one day at a time, and when people start giving you the attention you're not used to, remember that we are made in the image and likeness of God. Keep Him at the forefront of your mind and strive to remain humble because as quickly as we can gain attention, we can lose it.

One of the best quotes I like to use comes from Denzel Washington's role in the film *The Equalizer*. As he was helping a friend get in shape, he said, "Progress, not perfection." Those are the most important words to remember when rebranding ourselves.

Keys to remember:

1. Take responsibility for what you know.
2. Don't be afraid of the new you.
3. Stay humble
4. Keep God at the forefront.
5. Progress, NOT perfection.

CHAPTER 4

Are You Tired?

"Yes!" is my answer because..."

CHAPTER 4

Are You Tired?

"Yes!" is my answer because I am tired. I am tired of watching other people lose weight, tired of feeling like I'm being left behind, and tired of seeing everyone else with the correct mindset and motivation while I'm still just talking about it. I even became known for promoting health and fitness, which adds more pressure to the existing problem. Those who took shortcuts to lose weight don't bother me because that is not an option for me. I understand that in certain situations, it's a good option, but for me, reaching my goal will require determination, willpower, and dedication.

Seeing other people pass you up can be inspirational; however, on the flip side, when we know what we should be doing and aren't doing it, it feels like a slap in the face. And no one likes to be slapped, as far as I know. There is nothing more powerful than a made-up mind. So, as I embark on this journey to finally reach my goal of two hundred pounds this year, my fuel is that I AM TRULY TIRED. I want to ask you: Are you truly tired yet? Because once we reach that place, we will change our actions.

From the first day I decided to start losing weight, it felt like I was instantly enrolled in school all over again. The only difference this time is that GOD was the principal, LIFE was the teacher, and I, of course, was the student. To be a good student and do well on the test, we must take plenty of notes, ask plenty of questions, and pay attention in class. Each year has prepared me to handle reaching my desired weight properly because temptations will come from all directions, not just sexual. Our character may even be challenged.

I cannot stress enough the importance of keeping God at the forefront of our thinking as we pursue better health, fitness, and wellness. It will be and is our protection. A good indication that we have transformed our mindset is when we start seeing solutions rather than making excuses. Instead of finding reasons not to do something, we find a way to stay on track with our task. It doesn't matter what the task is—whether it's losing weight, finishing school, building a business, or fixing your marriage—once we reach the point where we are ready for real change, we will "FIGHT 4 LIFE" and remove all excuses to get the job done.

CHAPTER 5

Are You Serious?

"Each phase of this journey comes with..."

CHAPTER 5

Are You Serious?

Each phase of this journey comes with a question we must ask ourselves and answer with our actions. As time continues to tick and tock, many temptations come day after day. As you may know, it's easy to be strong in front of people, especially if we know they're watching us or might expose our weaknesses. Now that I have been working in transportation for the last ten years, I had to ask myself: Was I serious about losing weight and living a healthier lifestyle? At times, when no one was around, I would walk into a gas station to get some gas but walk out with chips, soda, taquitos, or whatever I wanted, thinking that the next exercise just had to be a little harder and a little longer to burn off that snack.

But most of the time, that workout never happens because tomorrow is not a day of the week like Sunday, Monday, Tuesday, Wednesday, Thursday, Friday, or Saturday. As long as I was putting my task off until tomorrow, this snack was between me and me only—at least, that's what I thought. People are always watching us; it doesn't matter if we're in the spotlight or not. Friends, family, and strangers are all watching.

Growing up, I was told that talking to ourselves with a response meant we were crazy. So, having a conversation with myself was a no-no. But it's strange because once I started having these real discussions with myself, the results showed up more and more. For clarity, I am talking about mental discussions—looking in the mirror and speaking out loud to myself about the choices I am making.

Maybe that's what you need to do because the eyes see everything but themselves until a mirror is placed before them.

There have been times when I'd be riding in the car, and I would tell myself I was not serious about losing weight and being more fit. If I were, the weight would be gone. I will never forget the value of these discussions with myself. One day, I walked into a gas station and saw these fresh-out-of-the-oven donuts looking at me and calling my name. Recalling the previous talks with myself, I stood there for a few minutes, looking through the glass at the glazed donut with a little extra icing on it. Although it was tempting, I can't lie; I was able to walk away.

I was excited. It was such a victory that I called my wife, shared what happened, took a photo of the losers of this round, and made a post on social media. At that moment, it became clear that keeping my word to myself was the most important key to losing weight. No one in the gas station knew me, my struggle, or my goal to lose weight. If I grabbed a dozen donuts, nobody would know but me. I realized that as long as it did not matter to me that I was not keeping my word to myself when no one was around, the victory would never be mine, and most importantly, my health would not improve either.

Keys to remember:

1. Having a Q&A with yourself aloud & mentally is okay.
2. When it matters to you, the results will show up.
3. Tomorrow is NOT a day of the week.

CHAPTER 6

Why Are You Holding Onto It?

"During the process of losing weight..."

CHAPTER 6

Why Are You Holding Onto It?

During the process of losing weight, our clothes size goes down, and we have to buy new clothes. Honestly, whether male or female, we all enjoy buying clothes, especially in smaller sizes. As mentioned before, the weight would fluctuate at the start of this process. Initially, I bought new shirts and pairs of pants here and there. Then, one day, I stopped buying new clothes and told myself that once I reached my goal, I could shop for new clothes. As time continued to tick and tock, it became clear to me that it was so easy to regain the weight because I was holding on to clothes that I should have been getting rid of.

Even when I bought smaller sizes for myself, the idea of getting rid of the larger clothes never crossed my mind. Subconsciously, I knew that I was not committed to losing the weight and keeping it off. This is an issue because it makes it easier to get off track. So, to those of you in this situation right now, go ahead and toss those large clothes away. Consider having a yard sale or donating them. Just get rid of them; it will force you to stay focused on the goal at hand.

One day, I was going through my clothes and realized I had all these clothes that were too big for me. I asked myself, "Why haven't you gotten rid of these clothes? What are you holding on to them for?" It was time to let go of the old me to make room for the new me to grow. As long as those clothes were present, I could "HIDE" the weight when it started coming back, and no one would notice because they had seen me wearing these clothes before.

To them, it was just a repeated outfit, right? It's not like people come up and check the size of your clothes. When I knew which friends would be around, I would wear something they had complimented me on the last time they saw me so it wouldn't be obvious that I was off track with my goal.

Once the clothes were gone, it was harder to let the weight come back because I would have nothing to wear if it did. Spending money on what you do not want is not a good feeling. Usually, we should kill our pride and ego, but it is not good when it comes to walking into the store to purchase a size you are striving to get away from. At times like that, let your pride and ego protect you from going backward and keep that fat away.

Keys to remember:

1. You're not fooling anybody.
2. Get rid of those clothes.
3. Let your pride and ego protect your progress (in a humble manner).

CHAPTER 7

What Is Your Why?

"During a conversation with one of my mentors, he stated..."

CHAPTER 7
What Is Your Why?

During a conversation with one of my mentors, he stated, "Your motives determine not only how you move but how far or if you move." Often, when it comes to losing weight, our motives are not to live a healthier lifestyle. Most of the time, we aim to look sexy. I'm sure you have heard the term "getting ready for the summer," right? Well, summer is only a few months out of the year—only a quarter of the year, to be exact. So, what happens after summer ends?

Bodybuilders can maintain that motivation because they get paid for it. However, you and I, for the most part, have another source of income. I remember reading an article about Usher. At the beginning of the article, it discussed his current workout routine, stating that he was riding a bike six miles to the gym to work out for a few hours and then riding the bike back home. As I read this article, I was amazed at what he was doing and started thinking that this was going to be my new routine and that this was what I had to do to get the results I wanted. But as I kept reading, I asked myself why this guy, already in shape and with a nice figure, was going so hard.

Later in the article, it stated that he was getting paid millions of dollars to play the role of a boxer in a film. That was his WHY. That was his motivation—he was getting paid to ride that bike six miles, spend half the day in the gym, and then ride back home after a hard workout. At that time, I laughed and said, "Can someone pay me a million dollars to lose weight? I could spend all day in the gym, not worry about work or bills, and focus on losing weight."

But that was not my reality, and it's not yours. So, what is your why? Is your why your children, your spouse, a friend, or yourself? Because if your why is weak, your input will be weak as well. Our why has to be something worth fighting for. When we are tired and want to give up, our why must fuel us to keep going during those times when no one is looking or able to work out with us.

So again, what is your why? What is your motivation? Do you want to live long enough to see your children have children? Would you like to run around the yard without losing your breath after a few seconds? Are you striving to get off some meds? Once we have a strong why, we will start to see the change in our actions, which will produce a change in our lives.

My why was weak, which allowed me to keep going up and down. Especially when the pressure came, my why couldn't hold me up. Now that my why has changed, it allows me to progress. It's giving me that fuel after a long day to go to the gym or to get up early after a long night and go to the gym. It gives me the strength to turn down food when I am not hungry, and most importantly, it keeps me on track when I am alone. So, I end this chapter asking you again: WHAT IS YOUR WHY?

Keys to remember:

1. Discover your why.
2. Make sure your why is bigger than you.
3. Select a WHY that can hold you up and refuel you.

CHAPTER 8

Who Knows?

"I remember when these words first came to me:
You cannot be..."

CHAPTER 8

Who Knows?

I remember when these words first came to me: "You cannot be successful without a team." That short sentence changed how I saw many things and introduced me to the importance of having a team around you that you can trust with your intimate goals. Holding ourselves accountable is essential, but having two, three, or five people hold you accountable to your goals increases your chances of accomplishing those tasks. If we are afraid to tell people we want to lose weight, we are not serious about it. Once our minds are made up to do something, we should not have a problem sharing it with the people close to us.

There was a time when my organization was having a juicing challenge, and we wanted to put the word out to everyone who could benefit from it. We used social media, tagged people, and promoted it in various ways. One day, I got a message from a person expressing that our approach was wrong and that we should not have put the juicing challenge on people's timelines and tagged them. They told me they were sensitive about their weight and knew they needed to lose weight. Honestly, I was shocked and didn't know what to say because our motive was to inspire people to learn the value of juicing, lose a few pounds, and have a chance to win money at the end of the challenge. Needless to say, they did not participate in the juicing challenge, which hurt me because they didn't see the value of it.

At that time, I realized that people are truly sensitive about their weight and that we are not always aware of how people see themselves or think about themselves. Growing up, I didn't play sports or go outside much—not because my family held me hostage, but because it wasn't on my mind. Playing games wasn't an option. I mostly sat with the elders, watched TV, or listened to what they shared about life and various topics. Having a nice body was not a thought in my mind for years. By the time I noticed that my stomach was starting to hang over my waistline, it was too late. I remember bragging to my cousin that I was big-boned, but my stomach was flat.

Life must have phases where we function unconsciously, and then we wake up one day realizing how much we have done or not done in our lives. It felt like I went from the little guy to the big guy overnight and couldn't figure out when the weight came. People started calling me "big guy," "fatboy," "the boy with man boobs," and other things that didn't make me feel good about myself. I understood how this person felt about their weight, but they didn't know I could relate. I wondered how far back their story went because mine went back to the seventh grade, maybe even the fifth.

Throughout life, there were many times when I would exercise in my room with the door closed because I didn't want anybody to know that I wanted to lose weight—not even my mom. I would work out alone, doing whatever exercises I knew then, which wasn't a lot. Fast forward to adulthood, and that same mentality still existed. There were times I told myself I wasn't going to tell anyone and that one day, I would just walk into a room, and people would see the new me, the skinny guy. But that day never came.

In fact, as I shared a few chapters back, the results didn't show up until I started letting people know that I was working on losing weight and needed help.

So, it touched me deeply because I knew where they were coming from. More importantly, I knew they had to overcome a few things before they could start to free themselves from that mental cage. That is exactly what it is—a mental cage that enslaves us from facing our reality. If you can relate, I encourage you to speak up and create an accountability team around you that will inspire you and hold you accountable for being the best you can be. Our power lays dormant inside us as long as we deny what bothers us. From my personal journey, I know this is true. Even writing this is proof enough. You might say there have been people bigger than me who wrote books, and you may be correct, but did they write about their desire to lose weight, or was their book on every subject but that?

Keys to remember:

1. Stop working alone and speak up.
2. It takes a team to be successful.
3. Conquer your fears and face your reality.

CHAPTER 9

Are You Ready?

"Are you ready?" is a question we cannot answer verbally; it must be answered through..."

CHAPTER 9
Are You Ready?

“Are you ready?” is a question we cannot answer verbally; it must be answered through our actions. We know the sayings "a picture is worth a thousand words" and "actions speak louder than words." That is how those watching will see that we are ready. Our actions and our results in getting the weight off and keeping it off say that we are ready more than us yelling it from the top of Mount Everest.

There is such a thing as talking too much about what we are doing or are about to do. Honestly, I personally think that when we keep talking about what we are about to do, it weakens us and our desire to get the task done, but that is my opinion. I have come to realize that only a few people need to know what you're working on so they can either support you or hold you accountable for getting the job done. There is no need to tell the world about your plans or goals. There are forces that we can prevent from coming against us by moving in the proper manner because there are rules to being successful in life, and they work. We don’t have to discover a new path to success.

I knew I was ready to get the weight off and keep it off when I started changing my eating habits, stopped missing workouts, started talking about my failures without shame, and, most importantly, began facing my weaknesses one at a time. Again, no one can tell you when you are ready—they can see it if they understand, and if they do, they know they cannot tell you. It’s like that saying: when the student is ready, the master will appear. They can agree with you, but a person cannot walk up to someone overweight and say,

"Yes, you're ready to lose weight." It just doesn't work like that. However, if you are having a discussion with them, and they understand where you are and can see where you are at, and during the conversation, you say, "I am serious about losing weight; I am ready now," at that time, the person can say, "YES, you are."

If you think about it, the steps taken to get off drugs or alcohol are the same steps for losing weight, especially the first step of realizing and accepting that we have a problem and understanding that this issue is hazardous to our well-being. If I can stress any point to those of you working on your health and wellness, it is to surround yourself with people who are heading in the same direction as you and those who are where you want to be. Yes, this falls under having a great team around you because, as the saying goes, "Show me the five people you spend most of your time with, and I'll show you your future."

Another thing I couldn't stress enough is to trust the process and be consistent with working on your task at hand because that is part of being ready to complete the goal. I recall a time when a group of my peers would always say they were about to do something. After a while, I gave them the name "the about to crew" because, for each goal they had, it was clear that they were not ready to accomplish them. They were always "about to do it" and not doing it already. They taught me that when we have an idea we're serious about, we will start moving toward it immediately. They also taught me that when we have an idea that we want to do but lack the confidence in ourselves to do it, we seek the approval of others and want them to do the work for us, allowing us to say we played a part in it.

The only way to build our confidence is by setting small goals and reaching them. Each time we do that, it builds us up so that when we have an idea that may seem far-fetched to our peers or even ourselves, we have some confidence to get it done, no matter who can see it. I say that if you have a circle of people who can't think big, why keep them around? Our loyalty should be to ourselves first because there is no one who can live out our dreams but us. So why continue to wait on others to understand where we are or where we desire to go? I dare you to think big. I dare you to attack your health and wellness full throttle. Don't repeat my failures; allow this work to be your cheat code to get to the end faster.

Keys to remember:

1. Trust the process.
2. Don't be afraid to share your shortcomings.
3. Realize the importance of being healthy and fit.
4. Accept the dare.

CHAPTER 10

Get it Off, Keep it Off

"Get it Off, Keep it Off" is all about letting go of the things that..."

CHAPTER 10

Get It Off, Keep It Off

"Get it Off, Keep it Off" is all about letting go of the things that weigh us down and hold us back. We will be surprised to realize that certain events in our lives have power over us; even though we may consider them things of the past, they remain more present than current issues in our lives. One way to identify these burdens is by introspection and asking tough questions to uncover unresolved situations. These could range from experiences like being touched in fifth grade to not making the basketball team. The mind is powerful, so it's crucial to liberate it from being controlled by our past and allow our present life to take precedence.

We control our brains, not vice versa. When it comes to our health, fitness, and well-being, we must take time to purge ourselves to function optimally at all times. Many of us are physically overweight in America, a known fact. However, we are also mentally burdened by past events, whether recent or decades old. It's time to unload this emotional baggage. The biggest challenge in getting rid of and keeping things off is admitting that something is bothering us. During my weight loss journey a few years ago, I had to ask myself tough questions about what was holding me back and why I hadn't addressed it.

As I searched for answers, many things became clear. I realized that we must first ask the right questions and be honest with ourselves to progress. Some of us may have less baggage than others, but we all have burdens. As long as we refuse to face them, we cannot lighten our mental load, which often manifests physically, leading to various illnesses.

Once Americans start shedding this weight, life will become more heavenly and less hellish. We live in a world where food, drugs, and alcohol are easily accessible. Sadly, many place more faith in these than in a higher power, exacerbating sickness. Until we confront our issues, we cannot overcome them.

As I observe people who seem to have given up on life, I realize they begin their days seeking highs they'll never attain again. This isn't why we're on Earth. So, if you struggle with shedding weight mentally or physically, take time to introspect. Identify the root of the issue and uproot it to grow to the next level. God made us in his image; he'd prefer us to be healthy rather than constantly unwell.

CHAPTER 11

A Slimmer You?

"I've learned many lessons about weight loss, from weighing over..."

CHAPTER 11

A Slimmer You

I've learned many lessons about weight loss, from weighing over 300 pounds to losing more than seventy. In this chapter, you'll learn four tips on dropping weight without feeling overwhelmed. Welcome to an opportunity to become a slimmer and healthier version of yourself. This short chapter offers information and guidance for individuals on any fitness level, even those with busy schedules. The effectiveness and simplicity of these four steps make them easily achievable. When reading each step, keep an open mind to avoid self-sabotage. Becoming slimmer is simpler than you think.

Step One: Cold Water

Drinking water can temporarily increase the body's metabolic rate, contributing to burning more calories throughout the day. This effect occurs because the body needs to expend energy (calories) to heat the water to body temperature.

Water is an effective appetite suppressant. Drinking water before meals can create a feeling of fullness, reducing calorie intake during the meal. Additionally, proper hydration helps distinguish between hunger and thirst signals, preventing overeating.

Proper hydration is essential for optimal fat metabolism. When dehydrated, the body may struggle to break down fat stores efficiently, hindering weight loss progress. Ensure adequate water intake to support fat metabolism effectively. Drinking water regularly is essential for your overall health.

Carrying a gallon-sized reusable water jug helps track daily water consumption. Drinking a gallon of cold water within twenty-four hours can be challenging, especially without measuring. Consider using a gallon-size container with motivational words for encouragement. To make drinking water more enjoyable, infuse it with fruits, vegetables, or herbs of your choice. Invite a friend to join you or create a game out of it.

Step Two: Walking

"Walking is the best exercise."

Elijah Muhammad

Entering a gym wasn't easy when I weighed over three hundred pounds. Instead, I found a park with a trail near my residence and started walking daily. I gradually increased my activity level, starting with a few laps and progressing to jogging. The key is to start where you are and gradually build up. Walking is a low-impact aerobic exercise that helps burn calories and contributes to weight management.

Incorporating regular walking sessions into your routine can create a calorie deficit, which is essential for weight loss. Walking strengthens the cardiovascular system, lowers blood pressure, and reduces the risk of heart disease and stroke. It also boosts mood and reduces stress, anxiety, and depression, promoting relaxation and mental well-being.

Create a walking schedule based on your availability, aiming for at least four to six days a week. Start small and gradually increase your walking distance. Remember to mix up your routes and track your progress.

Step Three: Get Your Rest

Establish a relaxing bedtime routine to signal to your body that it's time to wind down and prepare for sleep. Activities like reading, taking a warm bath, or practicing relaxation techniques can help promote restful sleep.

Tips for Better Sleep:

1. Practice stress management techniques to reduce stress levels.
2. Avoid consuming caffeine and alcohol close to bedtime.
3. Engage in regular physical activity to improve sleep quality.
4. Aim for at least 30 minutes of moderate-intensity exercise most days of the week. Find what works for you and prioritize quality sleep for overall well-being.

Step Four: No Eating Late

"The best time to eat is between 4-6 pm."

Elijah Muhammad

By making conscious choices about when and what you eat, practicing mindful eating, and avoiding late-night snacking, you can take control of your eating habits and support your weight loss goals. Remember, small changes can lead to significant results over time. Avoiding late-night eating can prevent weight gain and promote healthier habits.

Replace late-night snacks with a soothing cup of herbal tea. Choose caffeine-free varieties such as chamomile, peppermint, or lavender to promote relaxation and aid digestion.

Sipping herbal tea can satisfy cravings for warmth and comfort without adding extra calories. Aim to have balanced and satisfying meals earlier in the day to prevent excessive hunger and cravings later on.

Include a mix of protein, fiber, healthy fats, and complex carbohydrates to help keep you feeling full and satisfied for longer periods. Sometimes, thirst can be mistaken for hunger. Before reaching for a late-night snack, drink a glass of water to see if your cravings subside. Staying hydrated throughout the day can also help prevent excessive hunger and cravings.

Eating late at night can contribute to weight gain due to the extra calories consumed when the body is less active and less able to burn them off. Furthermore, late-night eating is often associated with consuming high-calorie, high-fat, and high-sugar foods, which can contribute to weight gain over time if consumed regularly. Additionally, late-night snacking can lead to mindless eating and overeating, as individuals may be less mindful of portion sizes and hunger cues. We must always stay in control of our health and wellness.

These are the four simple steps to drop the pounds and become a slimmer and healthier version of yourself. Start Now! The worst thing we can do after receiving new information is wait to see if it actually works for us unless we've already mastered these four simple steps to increase our chances of dropping the pounds and becoming a slimmer version of ourselves. Start applying these principles to your lifestyle and discover the best ways to succeed in your wellness journey. These steps have worked wonders for me along my journey, and I know how essential they are to shedding pounds and inches.

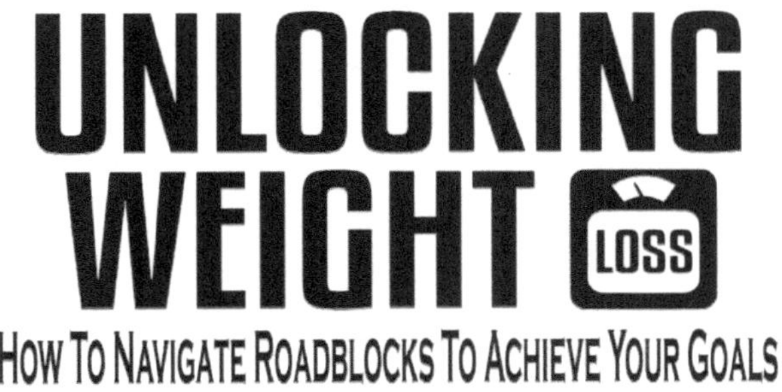

NOTES SECTION

NOTES

NOTES

NOTES

NOTES

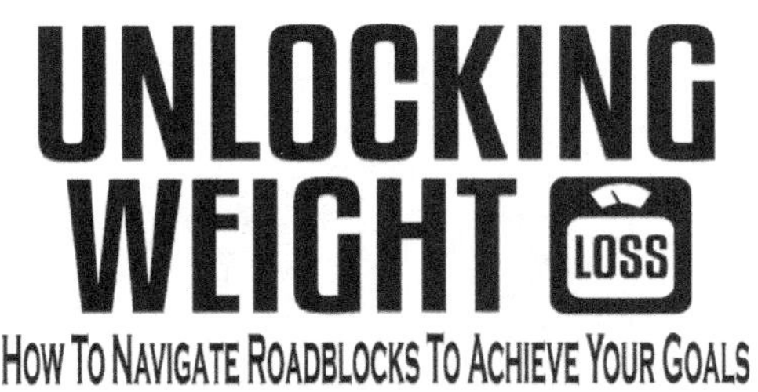

ABOUT THE AUTHOR

By: The Wellness Preacher

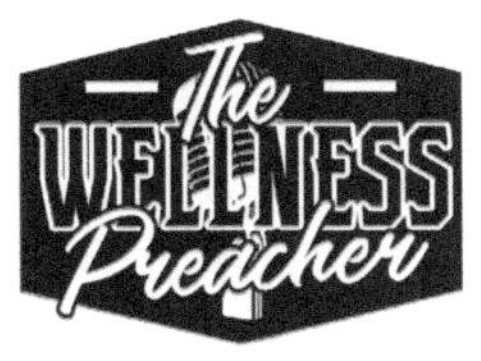

I am The Wellness Preacher

Your Brother & Servant

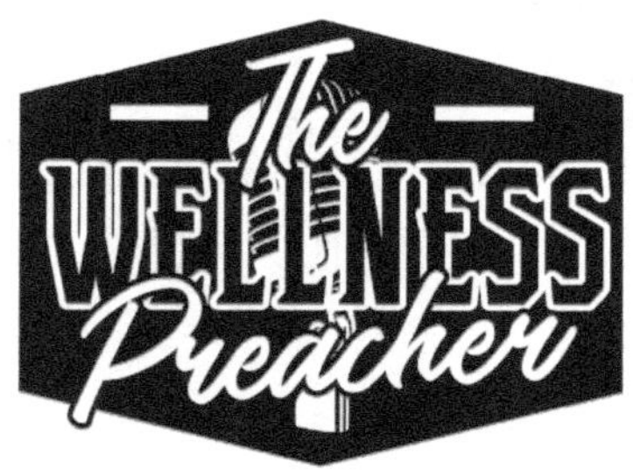

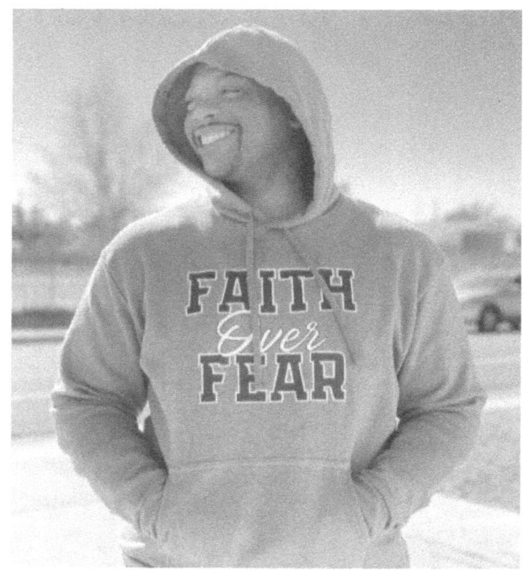

ABOUT THE WELLNESS PREACHER

The Wellness Preacher, also known as Brother Qaadir'Naqib Muhammad, was born in Pasadena, CA. At just 37 years of age, he has over twenty years of experience mentoring the generations coming behind him. Growing up in an environment infested with drugs and gang violence, with an absent father and a mother with an addiction, The Wellness Preacher was able to navigate through these circumstances. He avoided becoming a product of his environment and decided to change the narrative for his story.

He is the author and one of the founders of "Fight 4 Life" NO EXCUSES, a (501C3) non-profit organization that teaches life skills to young men between the ages of eight and seventeen. He has earned the name *The Wellness Preacher* from his passion for God, God's word, health and wellness, and his commitment to empowering humanity to do and be better inside and out. The Wellness Preacher is also a grandfather, father, husband, and he believes that family is business and business is family.

www.TheWellnessPreacher.com
IG: @thewellnesspreacher

OTHER BOOKS BY THE WELLNESS PREACHER

Breaking Mental Chains: Unlocking The 7 Mind Hacks

"Conquer your fears
& embrace your purpose."

The Wellness Preacher

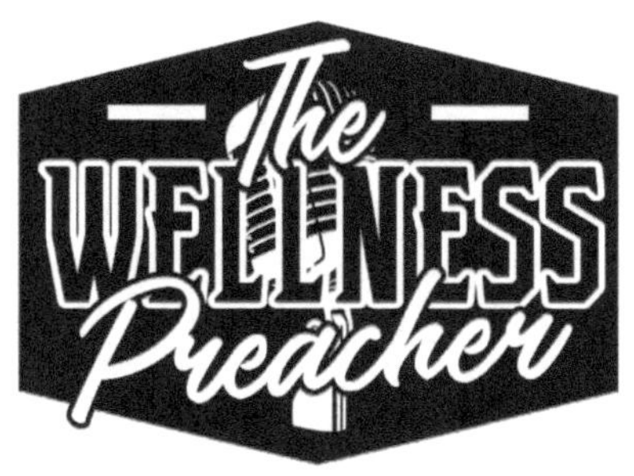

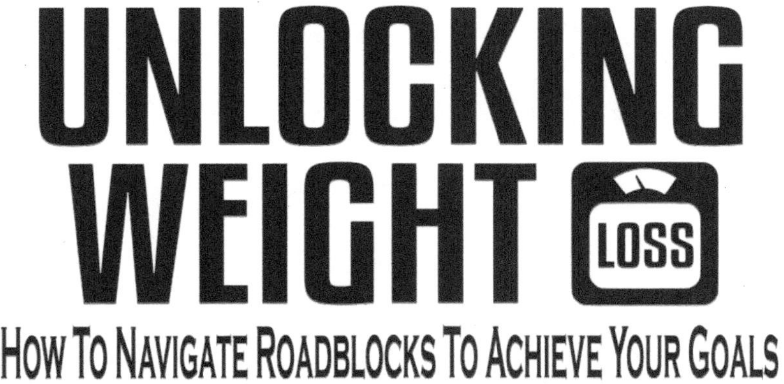
UNLOCKING
WEIGHT
LOSS
HOW TO NAVIGATE ROADBLOCKS TO ACHIEVE YOUR GOALS

www.ingramcontent.com/pod-product-compliance
Lightning Source LLC
LaVergne TN
LVHW090617110826
845146LV00001B/424

* 9 7 9 8 9 9 0 3 9 7 4 5 3 *